My Oily Everything Book

Helping the serious oiler keep all things oily in one convenient place.

MICHELLE L. HUDDLESTON

Hey Y'all!

If you are anything like me, you may have a binder, folder, notebook, and/or planner for everything and every area in your life. If you are not like me, you will still find this book totally necessary for all your oiling needs. Packed in this handy dandy book are easily accessible sections for every area of life. From inventory and must-try products to individual profiles and recipes, you'll be glad you purchased this book (or received it as a gift).

From one serious oiler to the next, I know how important it is to keep life as stress-free as possible. I'm a Wife, Mom, Mompreneur, homeschooling Mom, Chef, self-identified Nurse, Housekeeper... you get my point. I wear many hats, and something I have learned to do is use 100% pure, therapeutic-grade essential oils, and oil-infused products in each and every area of me and my family's life to help support the many systems and functions of our bodies.

Whether I'm soothing a boo-boo, cooking a "gourmet" meal, helping the kiddos focus on school work, or relaxing after an eventful day – I'm finding more and more ways to incorporate our oils and supplements. Now, instead of having papers, notebooks, and sticky notes all over the place... everything is conveniently kept in one place – *My Oily Everything Book.*

Where it's at...

Quick-Guide Charts

&

Carrier Oil Information

Take the guess work out of measuring your own blends with the easy-to-understand essential oils chart on the next page. The quick-reference carrier oil chart will also help when deciding what carrier oils are best for you and your family.

ESSENTIAL OIL DILUTION CHART

Dilution	1%	2%	3%	5%	10%	25%
Measurement of carrier oil.	Drops of essential oil per percentage.					
1 tsp, 1/6 oz, 5 ml	1	2	3	5	10	25
2 tsp, 1/3 oz, 10 ml	2	4	6	10	20	50
3 tsp, ½ oz, 15 ml	3	6	9	15	30	75
4 tsp, 2/3 oz, 20 ml	4	8	12	20	40	100
5 tsp, 5/6 oz, 25 ml	5	10	15	25	50	125
6 tsp, 1 oz, 30 ml	6	12	18	30	60	150

CARRIER OIL CHART

Skin Type	Oil Types		
	Liquid	Soft	Brittle
Normal	Grapeseed Sweet Almond	Coconut	Cocoa Butter
Oily	Grapeseed, Jojoba, Sweet Almond	-------	-------
Dry	Avocado, Olive,	Coconut	Cocoa Butter
Sensitive	Apricot Kernel, Sweet Almond	-------	-------
Mature	Grapeseed, Almond	Shea Butter	-------

Useful information: Some carrier oils are prone to clog pores more than others. Do a patch test before trying a new carrier oil.

Quick Guide Charts & Carrier Oil Information

Use this space to right down your own notes.

_____

_____

_____

_____

_____

_____

_____

_____

_____

_____

_____

_____

_____

_____

_____

_____

_____

Inventory

Use the following pages to keep track of what is in your essential oil, oil-infused product, and supplement inventory.

Some ways to get the most out of this section are:

- Use a pencil when writing for easy erasing and correcting.
- Write your products in alphabetical order to help easily locate them.
- Update as soon as you run out or order more of a product.
- Don't forget to document your accessories too (diffusers, diffuser jewelry, bottles, etc.).

A – C

Product	QTY	Product	QTY

D – G

Product	QTY	Product	QTY

H – J

Product	QTY	Product	QTY

K – M

Product	QTY	Product	QTY

N – P

Product	QTY	Product	QTY

Q – T

Product	QTY	Product	QTY

U – Z

Product	QTY	Product	QTY

NOTES

Accessories

Product	QTY	Product	QTY

Use this space to right down your own notes.

_____

_____

_____

_____

_____

_____

_____

_____

_____

_____

_____

_____

_____

_____

_____

_____

Budget
&
Get Lists

I know how important it is to budget. When it comes to purchasing your health and wellness products and accessories, it's no different than budgeting for groceries or a vacation.

Use these next several pages to set a monthly budget that you want to spend on purchasing your must-have and wanna-get products and accessories. Keep track of products that you need to re-order, as well as those you'd like to try. Write the prices next to the products for easy adding to ensure you don't go over budget! And, utilize the savings column to notate how much you save each month.

Tips and tricks to using this section:

- As always, I suggest you use a pencil for easy erasing, editing, and updating.
- Notate how much you spent to keep track of if you stayed below or went above budget.
- Arrange your list alphabetically, by need, or by price (low to high or high to low).
- Include free products and any cash/points-back programs when writing how much saved.

There are enough spaces to budget for 6 years.

Date	Budget	Spent	Saved
May 2017	*$100*	*$103*	*$30*

Budgeting Goals & Notes

_____

_____

_____

_____

_____

_____

_____

_____

_____

_____

_____

_____

_____

_____

_____

_____

Date	Budget	Spent	Saved
May 2017	*$100*	*$103*	*$30*

Budgeting Goals & Notes

_____

_____

_____

_____

_____

_____

_____

_____

_____

_____

_____

_____

_____

_____

_____

_____

Date	Budget	Spent	Saved
May 2017	*$100*	*$103*	*$30*

Budgeting Goals & Notes

_____

_____

_____

_____

_____

_____

_____

_____

_____

_____

_____

_____

_____

_____

_____

_____

Get list for essential oils.

Product	Cost	Date Purchased

Get list for essential oils.

Product	Cost	Date Purchased

Get list for oil-infused products (bath, body, oral care, etc.).

Product	Cost	Date Purchased

Get list for supplements.

Product	Cost	Date Purchased

Get list for accessories.

Product	Cost	Date Purchased

Individual

Oily

Profiles

Keep track of every family member's oily profile in a super convenient way (even pets)! Use this section to write down go-to oils, products, and recipes for every member in your household. Be sure to take note of oils and products that you want to avoid for each family as well.

Get the most from this section by noting special oily uses from oily bath and bedtime routines to your go-to blends for focusing and relaxing. There are enough pages for 10 family members.

Family Member: Trevor

Birthdate: April 28

. . . .

Most used oils, products, supplements, and accessories:

_____	_____
_____	_____
_____	_____
_____	_____
_____	_____
_____	_____

Oils, products, supplements, and accessories to avoid:

_____	_____
_____	_____
_____	_____
_____	_____
_____	_____

. . . .

Special care notes:

_____

_____

_____

_____

Special recipes, blends, and mixtures:

Used for: _Gout_

_____

_____

_____

Used for: _____

_____

_____

_____

Used for: _____

_____

_____

_____

Used for: _____

_____

_____

_____

Used for: _____

_____

_____

_____

Family Member: _____

Birthdate: _____

. . . .

Most used oils, products, supplements, and accessories:

_____   _____

_____   _____

_____   _____

_____   _____

_____   _____

_____   _____

Oils, products, supplements, and accessories to avoid:

_____   _____

_____   _____

_____   _____

_____   _____

_____   _____

. . . .

Special care notes:

_____

_____

_____

_____

Special recipes, blends, and mixtures:

Used for: _____

_____

_____

_____

Used for: _____

_____

_____

_____

Used for: _____

_____

_____

_____

Used for: _____

_____

_____

_____

Used for: _____

_____

_____

_____

Family Member: _____

Birthdate: _____

. . . .

Most used oils, products, supplements, and accessories:

_____   _____

_____   _____

_____   _____

_____   _____

_____   _____

_____   _____

Oils, products, supplements, and accessories to avoid:

_____   _____

_____   _____

_____   _____

_____   _____

_____   _____

. . . .

Special care notes:

_____

_____

_____

_____

Special recipes, blends, and mixtures:

Used for: _____

_____

_____

_____

Used for: _____

_____

_____

_____

Used for: _____

_____

_____

_____

Used for: _____

_____

_____

_____

Used for: _____

_____

_____

_____

Family Member: _____

Birthdate: _____

. . . .

Most used oils, products, supplements, and accessories:

_____   _____

_____   _____

_____   _____

_____   _____

_____   _____

_____   _____

Oils, products, supplements, and accessories to avoid:

_____   _____

_____   _____

_____   _____

_____   _____

_____   _____

. . . .

Special care notes:

_____

_____

_____

_____

Special recipes, blends, and mixtures:

Used for: _____

_____

_____

_____

Used for: _____

_____

_____

_____

Used for: _____

_____

_____

_____

Used for: _____

_____

_____

_____

Used for: _____

_____

_____

_____

Family Member: _____

Birthdate: _____

. . . .

Most used oils, products, supplements, and accessories:

_____   _____

_____   _____

_____   _____

_____   _____

_____   _____

_____   _____

Oils, products, supplements, and accessories to avoid:

_____   _____

_____   _____

_____   _____

_____   _____

_____   _____

. . . .

Special care notes:

_____

_____

_____

_____

Special recipes, blends, and mixtures:

Used for: _____

_____

_____

_____

Used for: _____

_____

_____

_____

Used for: _____

_____

_____

_____

Used for: _____

_____

_____

_____

Used for: _____

_____

_____

_____

Family Member: _____

Birthdate: _____

. . . .

Most used oils, products, supplements, and accessories:

_____   _____

_____   _____

_____   _____

_____   _____

_____   _____

_____   _____

Oils, products, supplements, and accessories to avoid:

_____   _____

_____   _____

_____   _____

_____   _____

_____   _____

. . . .

Special care notes:

_____

_____

_____

_____

Special recipes, blends, and mixtures:

Used for: _____

_____

_____

_____

Used for: _____

_____

_____

_____

Used for: _____

_____

_____

_____

Used for: _____

_____

_____

_____

Used for: _____

_____

_____

_____

Family Member: _____

Birthdate: _____

. . . .

Most used oils, products, supplements, and accessories:

_____	_____
_____	_____
_____	_____
_____	_____
_____	_____
_____	_____

Oils, products, supplements, and accessories to avoid:

_____	_____
_____	_____
_____	_____
_____	_____
_____	_____

. . . .

Special care notes:

_____

_____

_____

_____

Special recipes, blends, and mixtures:

Used for: _____

_____

_____

_____

Used for: _____

_____

_____

_____

Used for: _____

_____

_____

_____

Used for: _____

_____

_____

_____

Used for: _____

_____

_____

_____

Family Member: _____

Birthdate: _____

. . . .

Most used oils, products, supplements, and accessories:

_____   _____

_____   _____

_____   _____

_____   _____

_____   _____

_____   _____

Oils, products, supplements, and accessories to avoid:

_____   _____

_____   _____

_____   _____

_____   _____

_____   _____

. . . .

Special care notes:

_____

_____

_____

_____

Special recipes, blends, and mixtures:

Used for: _____

_____

_____

_____

Used for: _____

_____

_____

_____

Used for: _____

_____

_____

_____

Used for: _____

_____

_____

_____

Used for: _____

_____

_____

_____

Family Member: _____

Birthdate: _____

. . . .

Most used oils, products, supplements, and accessories:

_____   _____

_____   _____

_____   _____

_____   _____

_____   _____

_____   _____

Oils, products, supplements, and accessories to avoid:

_____   _____

_____   _____

_____   _____

_____   _____

_____   _____

. . . .

Special care notes:

_____

_____

_____

_____

Special recipes, blends, and mixtures:

Used for: _____

_____

_____

_____

Used for: _____

_____

_____

_____

Used for: _____

_____

_____

_____

Used for: _____

_____

_____

_____

Used for: _____

_____

_____

_____

Family Member: _____

Birthdate: _____

. . . .

Most used oils, products, supplements, and accessories:

_____   _____

_____   _____

_____   _____

_____   _____

_____   _____

_____   _____

Oils, products, supplements, and accessories to avoid:

_____   _____

_____   _____

_____   _____

_____   _____

_____   _____

. . . .

Special care notes:

_____

_____

_____

_____

Special recipes, blends, and mixtures:

Used for: _____

_____

_____

_____

Used for: _____

_____

_____

_____

Used for: _____

_____

_____

_____

Used for: _____

_____

_____

_____

Used for: _____

_____

_____

_____

Household Cleaning
& Cleansing

Put your favorite tips, tricks, and do-it-yourself cleaning hacks in this section. It is designed for you to note what supplies and products you need to have stocked in order to keep your home chemical-free. There is also a notes section to jot down places you purchase your supplies for easy re-ordering and/or gathering.

To give you an idea, most homemade products use the following ingredients: white vinegar, olive oil, borax, washing soda, baking soda, castile soap, and distilled water. The most commonly used essential oils are: lemon, orange, grapefruit, and lavender.

When making oil-infused products, it is suggested that you use a glass or BPA-free plastic container for storage. Ideas about where to purchase such products, and find easy recipes, can be found on the *Resources & References* pages at the end of this book.

Supplies to keep stocked:

_____   _____

_____   _____

_____   _____

_____   _____

_____   _____

_____   _____

Notes: _____

_____

_____

_____

Most commonly used essential oils:

_____   _____

_____   _____

_____   _____

_____   _____

_____   _____

_____   _____

Notes: _____

_____

_____

_____

Recipe for: _____

Ingredients & Measurements:

_____   _____

_____   _____

_____   _____

_____   _____

Instructions:

_____

_____

_____

_____

_____

Recipe for: _____

Ingredients & Measurements:

_____   _____

_____   _____

_____   _____

_____   _____

Instructions:

_____

_____

_____

_____

_____

Recipe for: _____

Ingredients & Measurements:

_____   _____

_____   _____

_____   _____

_____   _____

Instructions:

_____

_____

_____

_____

_____

Recipe for: _____

Ingredients & Measurements:

_____   _____

_____   _____

_____   _____

_____   _____

Instructions:

_____

_____

_____

_____

_____

Recipe for: _____

Ingredients & Measurements:

_____   _____

_____   _____

_____   _____

_____   _____

Instructions:

_____

_____

_____

_____

_____

Recipe for: _____

Ingredients & Measurements:

_____   _____

_____   _____

_____   _____

_____   _____

Instructions:

_____

_____

_____

_____

_____

Recipe for: _____

Ingredients & Measurements:

_____   _____

_____   _____

_____   _____

_____   _____

Instructions:

_____

_____

_____

_____

_____

Recipe for: _____

Ingredients & Measurements:

_____   _____

_____   _____

_____   _____

_____   _____

Instructions:

_____

_____

_____

_____

_____

Recipe for: _____

Ingredients & Measurements:

_____   _____

_____   _____

_____   _____

_____   _____

Instructions:

_____

_____

_____

_____

_____

Recipe for: _____

Ingredients & Measurements:

_____   _____

_____   _____

_____   _____

_____   _____

Instructions:

_____

_____

_____

_____

_____

Recipe for: _____

Ingredients & Measurements:

_____   _____

_____   _____

_____   _____

_____   _____

Instructions:

_____

_____

_____

_____

_____

Recipe for: _____

Ingredients & Measurements:

_____   _____

_____   _____

_____   _____

_____   _____

Instructions:

_____

_____

_____

_____

_____

What's Cooking?

Keep your favorite oil-infused recipes in one convenient place!

Recipe: _____

Category: _____

Servings: _____

Ingredients & Measurements:

_____ _____

_____ _____

_____ _____

_____ _____

_____ _____

_____ _____

Instructions:

_____

_____

_____

_____

_____

_____

_____

_____

_____

_____

_____

_____

_____

_____

Recipe: _____

Category: _____

Servings: _____

Ingredients & Measurements:

_____   _____

_____   _____

_____   _____

_____   _____

_____   _____

_____   _____

Instructions:

_____

_____

_____

_____

_____

_____

_____

_____

_____

_____

_____

_____

_____

_____

Recipe: _____

Category: _____

Servings: _____

Ingredients & Measurements:

_____   _____

_____   _____

_____   _____

_____   _____

_____   _____

_____   _____

Instructions:

_____

_____

_____

_____

_____

_____

_____

_____

_____

_____

_____

_____

_____

Recipe: _____

Category: _____

Servings: _____

Ingredients & Measurements:

_____   _____

_____   _____

_____   _____

_____   _____

_____   _____

_____   _____

Instructions:

_____

_____

_____

_____

_____

_____

_____

_____

_____

_____

_____

_____

_____

_____

_____

Recipe: _____

Category: _____

Servings: _____

Ingredients & Measurements:

_____   _____

_____   _____

_____   _____

_____   _____

_____   _____

_____   _____

Instructions:

_____

_____

_____

_____

_____

_____

_____

_____

_____

_____

_____

_____

_____

Recipe: _____

Category: _____

Servings: _____

Ingredients & Measurements:

_____   _____

_____   _____

_____   _____

_____   _____

_____   _____

_____   _____

Instructions:

_____

_____

_____

_____

_____

_____

_____

_____

_____

_____

_____

_____

_____

_____

_____

Recipe: _____

Category: _____

Servings: _____

Ingredients & Measurements:

_____   _____

_____   _____

_____   _____

_____   _____

_____   _____

_____   _____

Instructions:

_____

_____

_____

_____

_____

_____

_____

_____

_____

_____

_____

_____

_____

Recipe: _____

Category: _____

Servings: _____

Ingredients & Measurements:

_____   _____

_____   _____

_____   _____

_____   _____

_____   _____

_____   _____

Instructions:

_____

_____

_____

_____

_____

_____

_____

_____

_____

_____

_____

_____

_____

_____

Recipe: _____

Category: _____

Servings: _____

Ingredients & Measurements:

_____   _____

_____   _____

_____   _____

_____   _____

_____   _____

_____   _____

Instructions:

_____

_____

_____

_____

_____

_____

_____

_____

_____

_____

_____

_____

_____

_____

Recipe: _____

Category: _____

Servings: _____

Ingredients & Measurements:

_____   _____

_____   _____

_____   _____

_____   _____

_____   _____

_____   _____

Instructions:

_____

_____

_____

_____

_____

_____

_____

_____

_____

_____

_____

_____

_____

Recipe: _____

Category: _____

Servings: _____

Ingredients & Measurements:

_____   _____

_____   _____

_____   _____

_____   _____

_____   _____

_____   _____

Instructions:

_____

_____

_____

_____

_____

_____

_____

_____

_____

_____

_____

_____

_____

Recipe: _____

Category: _____

Servings: _____

Ingredients & Measurements:

_____   _____

_____   _____

_____   _____

_____   _____

_____   _____

_____   _____

Instructions:

_____

_____

_____

_____

_____

_____

_____

_____

_____

_____

_____

_____

_____

_____

Recipe: _____

Category: _____

Servings: _____

Ingredients & Measurements:

_____   _____

_____   _____

_____   _____

_____   _____

_____   _____

_____   _____

Instructions:

_____

_____

_____

_____

_____

_____

_____

_____

_____

_____

_____

_____

_____

_____

Recipe: _____

Category: _____

Servings: _____

Ingredients & Measurements:

_____   _____

_____   _____

_____   _____

_____   _____

_____   _____

_____   _____

Instructions:

_____

_____

_____

_____

_____

_____

_____

_____

_____

_____

_____

_____

_____

_____

Recipe: _____

Category: _____

Servings: _____

Ingredients & Measurements:

_____   _____

_____   _____

_____   _____

_____   _____

_____   _____

_____   _____

Instructions:

_____

_____

_____

_____

_____

_____

_____

_____

_____

_____

_____

_____

_____

_____

Recipe: _____

Category: _____

Servings: _____

Ingredients & Measurements:

_____   _____

_____   _____

_____   _____

_____   _____

_____   _____

_____   _____

Instructions:

_____

_____

_____

_____

_____

_____

_____

_____

_____

_____

_____

_____

_____

_____

_____

Recipe: _____

Category: _____

Servings: _____

Ingredients & Measurements:

_____   _____

_____   _____

_____   _____

_____   _____

_____   _____

_____   _____

Instructions:

_____

_____

_____

_____

_____

_____

_____

_____

_____

_____

_____

_____

_____

Recipe: _____

Category: _____

Servings: _____

Ingredients & Measurements:

_____   _____

_____   _____

_____   _____

_____   _____

_____   _____

_____   _____

Instructions:

_____

_____

_____

_____

_____

_____

_____

_____

_____

_____

_____

_____

_____

_____

Recipe: _____

Category: _____

Servings: _____

Ingredients & Measurements:

_____   _____

_____   _____

_____   _____

_____   _____

_____   _____

_____   _____

Instructions:

_____

_____

_____

_____

_____

_____

_____

_____

_____

_____

_____

_____

_____

_____

Recipe: _____

Category: _____

Servings: _____

Ingredients & Measurements:

_____   _____

_____   _____

_____   _____

_____   _____

_____   _____

_____   _____

Instructions:

_____

_____

_____

_____

_____

_____

_____

_____

_____

_____

_____

_____

_____

_____

The Great Outdoors

Whether you're camping, hanging out in the back yard, or spending the day at a ball park – the great outdoors can be both beautiful and pesky at the same time. Store all of your go-to outdoorsy recipes in this section.

Recipe for: _____

Ingredients & Measurements:

_____   _____

_____   _____

_____   _____

_____   _____

Instructions:

_____

_____

_____

_____

_____

Recipe for: _____

Ingredients & Measurements:

_____   _____

_____   _____

_____   _____

_____   _____

Instructions:

_____

_____

_____

_____

_____

Recipe for: _____

Ingredients & Measurements:

_____   _____

_____   _____

_____   _____

_____   _____

Instructions:

_____

_____

_____

_____

_____

Recipe for: _____

Ingredients & Measurements:

_____   _____

_____   _____

_____   _____

_____   _____

Instructions:

_____

_____

_____

_____

_____

Recipe for: _____

Ingredients & Measurements:

_____   _____

_____   _____

_____   _____

_____   _____

Instructions:

_____

_____

_____

_____

_____

Recipe for: _____

Ingredients & Measurements:

_____   _____

_____   _____

_____   _____

_____   _____

Instructions:

_____

_____

_____

_____

_____

Recipe for: _____

Ingredients & Measurements:

_____   _____

_____   _____

_____   _____

_____   _____

Instructions:

_____

_____

_____

_____

_____

Recipe for: _____

Ingredients & Measurements:

_____   _____

_____   _____

_____   _____

_____   _____

Instructions:

_____

_____

_____

_____

_____

Recipe for: _____

Ingredients & Measurements:

_____   _____

_____   _____

_____   _____

_____   _____

Instructions:

_____

_____

_____

_____

_____

Recipe for: _____

Ingredients & Measurements:

_____   _____

_____   _____

_____   _____

_____   _____

Instructions:

_____

_____

_____

_____

_____

Extra Notes

Extra Notes _____

_____

_____

_____

_____

_____

_____

_____

_____

_____

_____

_____

_____

_____

_____

_____

_____

_____

_____

_____

_____

Extra Notes _____

_____

_____

_____

_____

_____

_____

_____

_____

_____

_____

_____

_____

_____

_____

_____

_____

Resources & References

There are a wealth of resources and references that can help you along your health and wellness journey using 100% pure, therapeutic-grade essential oils and supplements. Some of my personal favorites are listed on the next page. Any that you find and want to remember, add them in the notes section.

Tips to consider while doing research:

- Ensure that your sources are credible and reliable.
- Unbiased resources and references offer great support.
- Double check advice given from others.

Books, brochures, glass bottles (spray and roller bottles), and accessories can all be purchased at Abundant Health 4 U (www.abundanthealth4u.com):

Reference Guide for Essential Oils (2017 edition) by Connie and Alan Higley

The Essential Home: A Companion to the Reference Guide for Essential Oils

The Chemical-Free Home by Melissa Poepping (there are also editions 2 & 3)

Essential Oils & Pets Booklet by Mary Hess

Life Science Products and publishing also has a wealth of resources. While they are geared toward a particular brand, majority of their books can be used by anyone (www.discoverlsp.com).

Essential Oils Desk Reference (also available as a pocket reference)

The Chemistry of Essential Oils Made Simply by Dr. David Stewart

Resources that can be found on Amazon

Gentle Babies by Debra Rayburn

Healing Oils of the Bible by Dr. David Stewart

French Aromatherapy: Essential Oil Recipes & Usage Guide by Jen O'Sullivan

Notes

Notes

Notes

Notes

Connect with Bryan & Michelle!

If you are interested in connecting with Bryan and Michelle, you can find them on the following social media spots:

Facebook: www.facebook.com/huddlestonfam

Instagram: in.this.life.of.ours

Email: essentialancientrememdies@gmail.com

Blog: www.essentialancientremedies.wordpress.com

Blessings on your lifestyle toward wellness, purpose, and abundance!

Made in the USA
Middletown, DE
03 April 2017